Better Eyesight without Glasses

BETTER EYESIGHT WITHOUT GLASSES

Dr CHINTHANA PATKAR
and
VIJAYA KUMAR

NEW DAWN PRESS, INC.
UK • USA • INDIA

NEW DAWN PRESS GROUP

Published by New Dawn Press Group
New Dawn Press, 2 Tintern Close, Slough, Berkshire, SL1-2TB, UK
e-mail: salesuk@newdawnpress.org

New Dawn Press, Inc., 244 South Randall Rd # 90, Elgin, IL 60123
e-mail: sales@newdawnpress.com

New Dawn Press (An Imprint of Sterling Publishers (P) Ltd.)
A-59, Okhla Industrial Area, Phase-II, New Delhi-110020
e-mail: info@sterlingpublishers.com
www.sterlingpublishers.com
www.newdawnpress.org

Better Eyesight without Glasses

ISBN 1 84557 444 3

PRINTED IN INDIA

Contents

Introduction

Of all our faculties, sight has consistently been considered the most miraculous and the most beneficial. Biology shows that the eye is, quite literally, a part of the brain, the place where the brain rises to the surface. Our eyes enable us to see things. But because of their complex mechanism, they are peculiarly liable to defect, breakdown and injury. Modern civilisation also places an unprecedented strain on the optic system of the ordinary person. Television screens, artificial lighting, abundant reading materials, poor diet, tobacco, alcohol, certain drugs, can all contribute to deteriorated vision.

This book is designed to provide the lay person with a comprehensive guide to how the eyes work, how to look after them, some easy-to-follow exercises for relaxation of the eye muscles, and better eyesight without glasses.

The Optics of the Eye

Sight can be the most informative of all the senses.

Our eyes constantly explore the world by scanning and inspecting the details of our surroundings. They adapt quickly to suit the surroundings. They can shift focus instantly in any direction, and their movements are rapid.

They adapt to the amount of light as well, letting in only that much as is required in bright sunlight but opening up to gather as much light as possible at night and in dim light.

External muscles of the eye

The eyeball is a slightly flattened sphere about an inch in diameter. It lies in a bony socket lined with fatty tissues, thus protecting the eye from any injury. Each eyeball is made up of three layers: the sclera, the choroid and the retina.

Sclera

This is the outer layer, consisting of a tough, protective tissue, which holds the eye in shape, and provides points of attachment for the external muscles that move it.

Behind the eyeball, the sclerotic layer is pierced by the optic nerve. The sclerotic tissue is opaque and normally white in colour. The visible part is covered with a transparent membrane called the conjunctiva which contains a network of tiny blood vessels that become enlarged if injured or inflamed, making the eyeball bloodshot.

There is a domed transparent window in front of the sclerotic layer, called the cornea, which lets light into the eye – one of the few tissues in the body having no blood vessels in them. Tears, one of the natural safeguards for the cornea, come from the lachrymal gland, behind the top eyelid, and drain into the narrow tear duct at the inner corner of the eye which leads to the back of the nose.

The tears, consisting of water containing salt and a bacteria-killing substance, spread over the cornea, and wash away the dust particles.

Choroid

The middle layer of the eyeball, the choroid, is dark brown or black, and the pigment absorbs excess light, thus preventing scattering of light in the eye and blurring of vision.

Many vessels, carrying blood and other fluids to the rest of the eye, pass through the choroid. The choroid, at the front of the eye, thickens to form a ring of muscle called the ciliary body which encircles the cornea. Ligaments attached to the ring hold the crystalline eye lens in its correct position. The lens can alter shape to complete the focusing.

The eyeball is divided into two chambers by the ligaments. The larger chamber, behind the lens, is filled with a transparent jelly, called vitreous humour, while the smaller one, in front of the lens, contains a watery liquid known as aqueous humour – both these fluids aid the eyeball in retaining its original shape.

The coloured part of the eye is the iris, which is also an extension of the choroid layer. It is suspended between the lens and the cornea. The circular opening at the centre of the iris is known as the pupil, which allows light into the eye. The iris automatically dilates and contracts the pupil to control the amount of light entering the eye.

Retina

The inner layer lining the back of the eyeball is called the retina.

This is a delicate, thin membrane whose surface is covered with a network of veins and arteries. Light travels through layers of nerve tissues underneath the retinal blood vessels before it reaches the light-sensitive receptors – the rods and the cones. The rods are slender and flat-ended, and the cones are thick and pointed. They are connected to nerve fibres that come together to form the optic nerve.

There are no visual receptors at this point, so it is not sensitive to light. It is known as the blind spot. It has no effect on vision because, when the eye is directed at something, its image falls on the central part of the retina, called the fovea.

The blind spot is in the field of the peripheral vision – the part seen out of the corner of the eye. The cones contain a violet pigment, and the rods a purple pigment, known as rhodopsin. When light strikes the rods and cones in the retina, chemical changes take place, resulting in bleaching of the pigments. Bleaching stimulates nerve signals that travel to the brain, where they are interpreted as a series of images. Bleaching occurs so quickly in the rods that they cannot operate in bright light – they are at their best in dim light, registering shades of grey, or at night when they can detect faint light sources.

The cones increase in concentration towards the back of the retina. In the centre of this area lies the fovea, a depression in which there are no rods, only cones. This is the area of sharpest vision, the point upon which light rays are focused when the eye is directed towards a particular point on an object.

It is sensitive to fine details because each of the cones is connected to a single nerve fibre conveying an impulse to the brain.

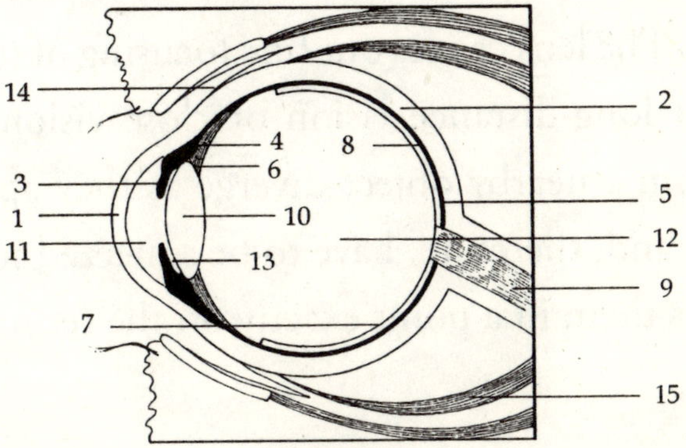

Figure 1

1. Cornea
2. Sclera
3. Iris
4. Ciliary muscle
5. Choroid
6. Suspensory ligaments
7. Retina
8. Fovea
9. Optic nerve
10. Lens
11. Aqueous (anterior chamber)
12. Vitreous (posterior segment)
13. Aqueous (posterior chamber)
14. Conjunctiva
15. Eye muscle

Refraction and focusing

When the light enters the eyeball, it is bent, or refracted. It passes through the conjunctiva, the cornea, the aqueous humour, the lens and the vitreous humour, before reaching the retina.

About 70 per cent of refraction takes place in the cornea. The lens carries out fine focusing of the light rays for long-distance vision or close vision. Light rays from a nearby object diverge as they approach the eye and, therefore, have to be squeezed together to focus them in a point exactly on the retina.

Light rays from a distant light source are almost parallel and so do not have to be refracted to the same degree.

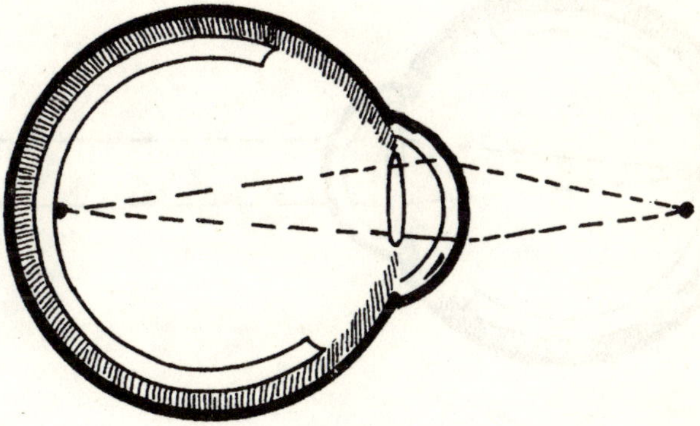

Figure 2

The ciliary muscle is the focusing mechanism of the eye, and it controls the suspensory ligaments and the shape of the lens.

When the ciliary muscle is relaxed, the lens flattens and rays of light from distant objects are sharply focused on the retina. For nearer objects, the ciliary muscle contracts to make the lens more curved and more powerful, thereby keeping the image on the retina in focus.

When the object is extremely close, its image goes out of focus and appears blurred. With age, the point of blurring changes as the lens gradually becomes stiffer and cannot change its shape so well.

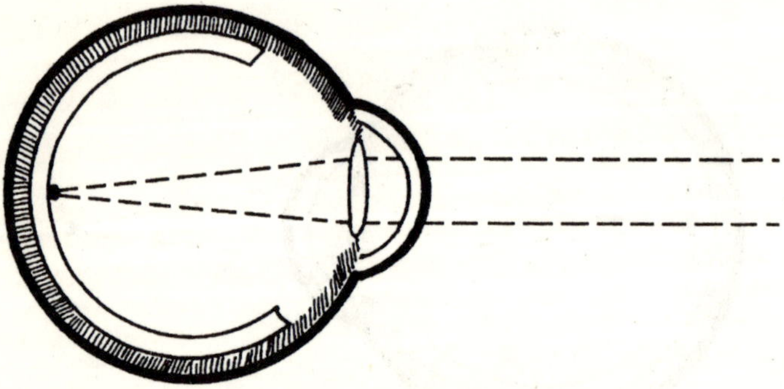

Figure 3

Three-dimensional vision

The brain and the eyes collaborate to give a three-dimensional image of the world. The two retinas receive tiny upside-down images of an object or scene. For objects about 20 feet or nearer, each retina has a slightly different, flat, two-dimensional view, and the difference in views is known as visual disparity.

The separate views from each eye reach the brain, where only the acceptable parts are instantly reassembled into a new picture – life-size and three-dimensional, having depth, height and breadth.

For objects beyond 20 feet, we use our memory of a familiar object to gauge the size of distant ones, and then the brain can judge the size of objects around a person. The way in which an object is placed in a scene influences our impression of size. The eye muscle also gives us information about distances – if an object can be seen clearly without conscious focusing, it is considered to be far away; if it can be seen with normal focusing, it is assumed to be nearby.

Sight and stability

When the gaze is fixed on a moving object, the eyes are held still, and the image of the object moves across the retina triggering signals in all the receptors in its path, thus giving information about the movement.

When the eyes move constantly, and the world around us appears to remain still, this sense of stability in visual experience is provided by the brain. Its commands cancel out the retinal movement signals.

As a consequence of this, when the eye tracks a moving object, its image remains stationary.

Cones and colour

It is believed that colour is analysed in the retina by receptor cells called cones.

There are three types of cones, each sensitive to one of the primary colours of light – red, green and yellow, and other colours are seen as combinations of these.

Anyone having a defective colour vision suffers from what is called colour blindness, the most common confusion being between red and green. A person may lack cones for one colour, or even two, and in very rare cases, all three colours.

Basics of Normal Vision

External features of the eyes

The outer parts of the eyes are protected by the eyebrows, eyelids and eyelashes.

Eyebrows, a line of short hairs growing on a bony ridge and covered with a thickened fold of skin, soaks up moisture, preventing it from running into the eye, shields the eye from sunlight and helps to protect it from blows.

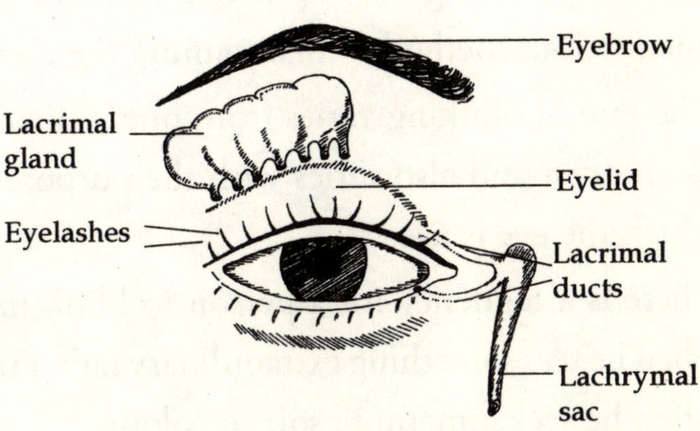

Figure 4

The eyelids are two folds of skin and tissue which can be closed with the help of the muscles to protect the eyeballs from excessive light or injury, and in blinking they form a film of antiseptic tears over the eyes.

The eyelashes form a fringe of stiff hairs protruding from the eyelids that brush away particles which might become lodged in the eye. Certain fundamentals, essential for normal vision, are blinking, flashing and shifting.

Blinking

- It is a quick, light, easy closing and opening of the eye, done intermittently by every normal eye.
- Nature has endowed us with eyelids, and their use in blinking is the most natural and unconscious method of maintaining the eyes.
- The rate of blinking varies from one individual to another, and also varies with the purpose for which the eye is used.
- There is a tendency for a person to blink more when he sees something extraordinary rather than when he sees something soft in colour.

- It is essential to keep the eyes moist, and blinking helps the lachrymal gland to produce the fluid to wash down and over the eyeball to keep it moist.
- The fluid has an antiseptic and cleansing quality.
- The eyes owe their brilliance and their ability to reflect light largely to the moisture.
- Since the cornea has no blood vessels, it requires this fluid to keep it moist, else it might result in corneal ulcers.
- When foreign particles enter the eye, the lachrymal fluids help in washing them out, and blinking in such cases releases more fluid.
- Frequent blinking of the eyes in winter tends to keep them warm.
- During stormy or dry weather, blinking protects the eye – it is better to blink more often as fluid is lost rapidly.
- The muscles of the pupil relax momentarily from tension between blinks.
- Blinking exercises the recti muscles, which is essential for their well-being.

- Blinking also helps in the circulation of the lymphatic fluid around the eye, thus giving strength to the eye.
- Any interference with blinking allows collection of dust which tends to induce inflammation of the cornea.
- Blinking acts as a shutter to intercept the rays of light entering the eye, and so preventing over-exposure of the sensitive receptive apparatus of the retina.
- Insufficient blinking and shutting of the eyes is the main cause for eye-strain and other sequential disorders.
- The eyes should blink quite freely and unconsciously.
- During constant nervous tensions, the eyelids remain open for long periods without blinking, instead of closing in easy relaxation, thus causing eye-strain.
- Deep in thought, one might stare at something unconsciously, leading to over-exposure.
- The permanency of good sight depends mostly upon the use of correctly acquired habits.

- The instinctive reaction of most people to a sound is that they turn their eyes or head to look for it though it is not visible.
- This action often becomes a fixed habit that most spectacled persons admit that they cannot hear nearly so well when they are not wearing their glasses. Frequent blinking and closing of the eyes ensures that the eyes are relieved of any kind of strain.
- For those wearing glasses, there is a necessity to keep the focus directed to the front and centre, in order to avoid the distortion that appears on looking to the side of the lens, thereby losing some of the muscular flexibility.
- When a person or patient is asked to keep his eyes closed more often for relaxation, it might interfere with his work, and also make him look somewhat conspicuous, especially during a meeting or a gathering. But the normal habit of blinking is free of such encumbrances, and in fact helps the routine by preventing strain and tiredness.

- The frequency of the visual impressions the eye makes is between thirty and forty images per second in an average person.
- Blinking increases the actual amount of time you may actively see, because failing to blink reduces the number of images to twenty or few images per second.

Flexibility

- For those who wish to establish normal vision, ensure that you are not only able to blink easily, but also habitually.
- See how quickly you can blink 20 times continuously without feeling the strain.
- If you find a break in rhythm, set about cultivating an easy flexibility by constantly blinking.
- In such cases, do not try to overcome many years' habit in a few minutes, but try to coax and encourage this blinking habit in a phased manner.
- If the eyelids are not as flexible as they should be, try this exercise: close your eyes tightly, exercising your muscles, then open them widely. Repeat this

five times, and try to do this exercise preferably every waking hour.

- In between these hours of exercises, practise easy, slow and deliberate blinking, beginning with five times at one-second intervals, and gradually increasing the number of consecutive blinks as flexibility is reached.
- Never practise rapid blinking until you have acquired the easy habit of slow blinking.
- While practising blinking, make sure that the eyes are wide open.

Flashing

- Look straight at the object you wish to see.
- Blink twice or thrice very quickly, regard the object for three seconds only, and at once shut the eyes, resisting the tendency of absorbing too much.
- Keep the eyes shut for a few seconds until they are relaxed and ready to see again.
- Open your eyes and repeat the blinking process, observe for three seconds again and close the eyes.

Shifting

- Shifting is a normal function and is normally done unconsciously.
- Shifting is both voluntary and involuntary in character.
- Shifting voluntarily is the movement of the eyes by will, from one point to another.
- The involuntary shift is continuous, automatic and very slight.
- Shifting should be as frequent as possible to exercise the eye muscles.
- An image takes about $^{1}/_{50}$ of a second to register on the retina, and this facilitates greater frequency of shifting with no loss of interruption of vision.
- Practise frequent shifting of the eyeballs in the following manner: remove your glasses, look at a word, then look at a couple of words beyond it, then back at the first word, and so on. Repeat this until the words become clear, relaxing as you practise. This constant shifting helps exercise the eye muscles.
- If you have good, normal vision, look at the moon, blinking frequently, shift your vision from

one end to the other end of the moon. Repeated shifting movements will make the moon stand out more clearly, making it appear as a truly solid body instead of a flat disc.

- The involuntary shift that is continuous is not visible, and corresponds in frequency with the rate of image produced in the retina.
- When one regards a large area, the eye makes a large and visible muscular movement from one part to another, the movement of the eyeball being natural in these conditions.
- By focusing on a smaller area, there is a tendency to keep the eye more or less fixed in focus since everything that one wants to view is within the range of the eye, making muscular movement unnecessary, and thus leading to strain.
- In such a case, there is a need to move the focus continuously even though the area is small.
- An exercise that helps in shifting focus is to use two or more objects of the same pattern and colour, placed at varying distances. Absorb the details of an object that is easily visible, then shift to another, absorb its details, and then shift to

the third object. By seeing clearly the detail and colour of the first object, you will be able to see the same detail and colour in the other two objects.

- When the eye is relaxed, the voluntary shifting is frequent but short in range.
- It is essential to have fine and well-trained movements of the eyeballs for the muscles to relax.

Alternate focus

- To enhance the flexibility of the eye muscles, consciously alternate the focus from a nearby point to a distant one.
- Hold up a finger fifteen inches from the face, in line with the eyes. Look clearly at the finger. Switch the focus in the same direct line to some other object beyond this – you will notice that while focusing in the distance, there seem to be two shadowy fingers. Then turn the focus back to the finger and repeat the process again.
- Similarly, standing near a window and looking at a spot on the window, then switching to

something outside the window at a distance, helps the muscles gain flexibility.

- These exercises can be done with each eye separately a few times before doing them together, for maximum benefits.
- This will be especially beneficial to those who spend a lot of time reading and strain their eyes.
- Even seeing the seconds hand of a watch move, for a few moment, also has its benefits.

Central Fixation

The retina has a small circular elevation in the middle which is 2 mm in diameter, called the macula lutea, derived from the yellow colour which it assumes in death.

In the centre of this macular area is a tiny depression known as the fovea which is the point of maximum sensitiveness. From the fovea, every other part is less sensitive in proportion to its distance, until at its extreme edge, the periphery where it is normally impossible to obtain acute vision. In the centre of the fovea there are only cones, not rods, which are elongated and pressed closely together.

Central fixation implies that the macular is normally so developed as to focus there, by virtue of its acutely developed receptive faculty.

In infants, during the first three weeks of life, the appropriate stimulus would normally develop the macular sensitiveness – a congenital disease during this period will result in the eye being unable later to hold or fix, a given object. Sometimes, later in life, due to various causes, the sensitiveness of the macula deteriorates, and is unable to hold or fix an object, resulting in an involuntary oscillatory movement of the eyeball known as nystagmus.

When one is able to focus a clear image of an object seen into the comparatively small area of the macula, one sees clearly, easily and effortlessly, since only the nerve-ends of acute vision are correctly stimulated. For those having myopia (short sightedness), hypermetropia (long sightedness) or astigmatism, the image is focused irregularly, and over a larger area, as a result of which the nerve-ends outside the macular area, though stimulated, do not have the required sensitiveness to respond, resulting obviously in a strain.

The strain is not only of local application, but to get the image of the object in its entirety. Instead of the visual centre in the brain being used to get a clear image, it has confused stimuli from other nerve-ends also, leading to visual blurring and mental aberration.

The nearer we habitually and consciously focus to a mathematical point, the less tired and strained will the eye be, provided the point of focus is kept moving.

Only a small amount of the whole range of vision is seen clearly at once, this small amount corresponding to the area of the image which falls only upon the macula.

The following diagram illustrates how only a relatively small amount, out of the whole area of vision, is seen clearly at one focus.

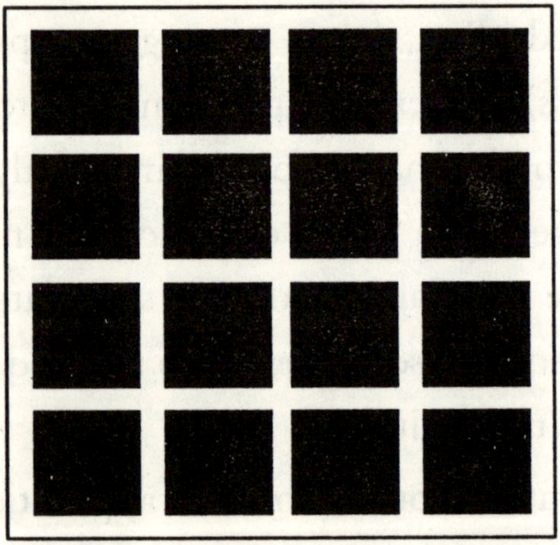

Figure 5

When you try to see the whole block in one focus, you will see a noticeable black shadow effect at each intersection of the white lines, but by focusing only on one black square, the shadow disappears. The fact that it is this constant and unceasing shifting of the small point of focus which is the mainstay of normal sight, cannot be overstressed.

When you are watching a film, try to see with macular vision, moving the focus from point to point, frequently blinking to counteract the tendency to stare.

The normal eye, besides seeing a comparatively minute point very clearly and the rest of the field less distinctly, changes that minute point of focus so rapidly and continuously that it is normally quite an unconscious action. The oculist assumes that refractive error is responsible for eye strain, and accordingly prescribes glasses to correct the error, little realising that it is the strain that produces the refractive error.

It is essential that those with normal sight maintain macular vision, while those with defective sight cultivate the habit of macular vision, for eyes seeing in this manner have better sight, with freedom from strain.

The cultivation of the habit can be done at any time and in any place, and never under pressure or force.

Exercise 1

- Hold a brightly coloured ball in each hand, both at arms length in front of you, about two feet apart.
- Looking directly at the ball in the left hand, observe in detail by moving the focus over it in any direction, and blink at least once every five seconds.
- You will be aware of the ball in your right hand, but do not look at it directly, for although visible as it is in the field of vision, it will not be clear in detail.
- Now repeat this process with the ball in the right hand.
- When you are confident of noticing the details of the ball in either one hand, bring the balls nearer till they are six inches apart.
- Repeat the same process of watching one ball at a time, till you see either one better than the other.

- Now bring the balls together till they touch together, and repeat the above process of watching one ball at a time.

Exercise 2

- Place a large chart illustrating large text letters, focusing good light upon it.
- Stand as far away as you can from the chart, and still are able to clearly see the large letters 'R' and 'B'.
- Close your eyes for a second or two and let them relax.
- Look quickly at the letter 'R' for a second only, and close your eyes again, realising that only that letter is clear, though the other is visible at the periphery of the eye.
- Repeat this exercise until you feel you can ignore the other letters, and see 'R' more clearly than anything else.
- Repeat this process with the letter 'B' next to 'R', keeping the glance to one second duration.

Exercise 3

- Move closer to the chart till you are two feet from it.

C	50 ft.
R B	25 ft.
T F P	18 ft.
5 C G O	14 ft.
4 K B E R	10 ft.
3 V Y F P T	8 ft.
2 Q C O G D C	5 ft.
R Z 3 B 8 S H F H O	4 ft.

Figure 6

- Look at the same letter 'B', and notice the three horizontal lines of the letter B – top, middle and bottom.
- Look at the top bar of the letter, and shift focus from one end to the other, observing the sharp, clearcut outline at the edges.
- As you observe the top bar, you will realise that it is clearer than the other two bars.
- Shift to the middle bar, and similarly notice that the other two bars are not so clear as the middle one.
- Practise this with the bottom bar, and you will realise that it is clearer than the other two.

Exercise 4

- Now stand in front of the chart so that the letters (10 feet) are visible but not quite clear.
- Close and relax your eyes.
- Open them briefly to notice only one letter on the line, and close the eyes quickly.
- Repeat this alternate flashing and closing of the eyes, with each eye separately, and then together, till this letter stands out clearer than the others.

- With this practice, you will soon realise that the period of clear vision obtained at first will gradually lengthen.

Exercise 5

- Another exercise for macular vision is the use of an ordinary clock face.
- Start with being close enough to see the numerals clearly.
- See a particular numeral while ignoring the rest till you can see it very clearly.
- Gradually increase the distance to as far as possible, but be sure to be able to distinguish one numeral clearly.
- With this exercise it becomes possible to lengthen the vision of sight.

Exercise 6

- Take a conveniently sized card, and make a circular hole in the centre, about 15 mm in diameter.
- Hold it flat against the reading matter, and move it along, so that you read only what is visible through the hole.

- Take care to blink frequently.
- Also alternate the use of each eye separately for a few lines, followed by both eyes together.

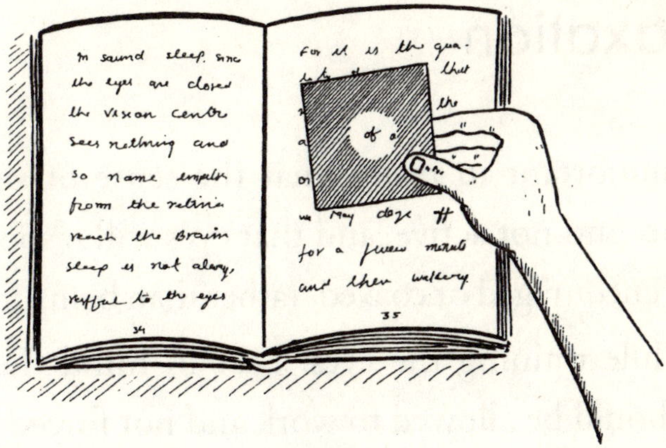

Figure 7

- It is usually better and easier to acquire macular vision on smaller letters than large ones, as the latter obtrudes the form of easily readable letters all at once on the field of vision, leading to eyestrain.
- It is better to frequently change one eye to the other rather than exercising one eye in particular for a long time.

Relaxation

It is important to realise that the sense of sight is passive, and not active, and that eyes will respond to being encouraged or coaxed, rather than being forced.

While training the eyes, bear in mind that the eyes should be allowed to work and not forced to do anything. The saying, 'let the light within you shine' aptly suggests how you should let the light within you, both spiritual and physical, manifest itself naturally.

Since we are continually stressed physically, mentally, emotionally or visually, we never allow the real light of truth to shine in its full capacity, but set up strains to distort the vision, whether optical or otherwise. Habitual and unnecessary strain leads to bad sight and bad health, especially astigmatism.

The greatest mistake made by most of us is to wait for an opportunity to relax, for the special opportunity does not present itself frequently, and may even be too late. Try to unload the strain throughout the day, without nervous pressure. Just relax in any way possible – sit down, close your eyes, think about something pleasant, take a few deep breaths.

Take out some time anytime during the day to stretch both your arms above your head, while simultaneously raising your eyebrows too for a few seconds half a dozen times. It would be well to remember that all phases of relaxation are purely passive, because relaxation can be combined with action and yet be quite free from stress and strain. Any form of fatigue, physical, emotional or mental, has a very quick and corresponding reaction upon the eyes which show the first symptom of tiredness.

This very first warning by the eyes must be heeded by allowing the body to relax completely, the mind to become calm, and the eyes to rest.

There are certain ways to logically and sensibly tackle fatigue as discussed below.

Sleep

In sound sleep, since the eyes are closed, the vision centre sees nothing, and so nerve impulses from the retina reach the brain.

Sleep is not always restful to the eyes, for it is the quality of sleep that matters more than the amount of sleep one gets. Sometimes we may doze off for a few minutes, and then wake up feeling refreshed – this is the sort of relaxation that the body and the eyes require rather than going to bed, laden with mental strains, nagging thoughts and doubts. The only way of easing off strain during the day is to cultivate the habit of freeing ourselves of it during the day, so that the mind is relaxed when retiring to bed.

The best way of inducing sleep is to lie comfortably on the back, with one hand on the chest and the other on the abdomen, breathing normally, but rhythmically by raising and lowering the abdomen.

Concentration

Concentration is the quiet exclusion of the inessentials, rather than straining to focus on a subject.

Singleness of purpose is essential for easy concentration. Real concentration should not be associated with fixation, strain, effort or rigidity. Since nothing in nature is rigid, we too need to cultivate the natural habit of shifting the focus continually.

Worry, fear and anxiety

Worry, fear and anxiety inevitably lead to nervous and mental disorders, and also eye-strain. The primary cause of eyestrain is not due to the amount of work they do, rather it is due to the way the work is done.

We have to face life as it actually is at present, and not as we fear it may become in the future – so face it with equanimity and joy instead of worrying unnecessarily. This frame of mind helps the eyes to function in a relaxed way, for your eyes always reflect your inner feelings.

Many people wish they could stop thinking too much, but they are not really thinking at all. Such people need to indulge in cheerful games and exercises which help to promote quick decision and this is reflected in their eyes.

Laughter and humour

The psychological value of humour is enormous and can scarcely be overrated. Even its outward expression in laughter form is like a breath of fresh air, and is most valuable in its physical reaction.

Nothing gives such a quickfire and valuable reaction to the eyes as a spontaneous response to the sense of humour.

Palming

It is essential for all of us, as we keep growing older, to apportion a certain period of the time to special ways of relaxing the eyes for longer periods.

Most people feel that by closing the eyes, it is much easier to rest and relax as the visual impacts are shut off. But mere closing of the eyes does not keep out all light. For example, we are able to determine whether we are in a lighted or a dark room. In order to totally relax the eyes, all light must be excluded which is done by palming.

Palming is a method of shutting out light by cupping the palms over the eyes so as to avoid pressure on the eyeballs.

With the palms cupped over the eyes, the fingers adjusted over the bridge of the nose, the eyebrows, and on the bony parts of the face and forehead, the elbows should rest upon a fairly firm cushion on the lap, or on a table or some other support to gain maximum relaxation. With light completely shut out, we are left with our thoughts or mental images, and an opportunity of utmost value to have one of the three powerful relaxants: physical relaxation, mental relaxation and visual relaxation.

Total relaxation is not possible if one of these relaxants is at fault, and hence palming is of utmost importance when it is done correctly. It is also essential that while palming is being exercised, the thoughts that one is left with should be pleasant, and not worried ones. Though all of us do have troublesome thoughts, it is better at any rate to leave them aside at least for those few minutes whilst palming.

When you find it difficult to control your worrisome thoughts, try to indulge in some pleasant thoughts of happy incidents in your life – your childhood memories, a memorable visit to some place, some exciting event, etc.

While you are letting your imagination roam, forget all about your eyes or palming. The duration of palming depends on each individual – one might like to do it for long periods, while another might get bored easily, and would like to do shorter stints at frequent intervals.

While occupying oneself with thoughts of something pleasant, ensure that you remember something familiar rather than wracking your brains to recall some vague memory whereby you are straining your mind. Many people claim that while palming, they are conscious of a changing range of colours which they believe to be some kind of supersense of light, but this is a sure sign of mental or emotional strain, for this is a condition of the eye which prevents a person from seeing black perfectly. The longer some people palm, the greater the relaxation they obtain, and the darker the shade of black they are able to see and remember.

Some people like to see colours while palming, and for such an exercise, take colour balls of equal size, one for each colour of the spectrum, against a black background. Picture each ball (following the order of the spectrum – red, orange, yellow, green, blue, indigo, violet) one at a time, giving the mind a clear impression of each colour, and soon you will find the black background standing out vividly against the colour ball. This shows that palming is a successful and one of the best methods of securing relaxation. If you palm perfectly, when you open your eyes, you retain all the relaxation that you have gained, and you do not lose it again.

Another exercise to achieve total relaxation is as follows: cover a table with a cloth of your favourite colour. Take a glance at it, and palm your eyes. Take occasional glances at the colour until you have a clear picture of it. While palming one eye, and keeping the other eye shut, use your free hand to roll a small ball around the table, following the movements of the ball in your mind.

This exercise can be varied by using different coloured back-grounds and using other objects instead of a ball. This exercise helps not only in directing the thoughts upon forms rather than abstract ideas, but also in the useful practice of shifting the point of focus continually. Picture one of the straight-lined letters like E or F on a chart. While palming, visualise each corner of the letter in sequence, noting each corner clearly and counting them as you proceed. Before finally opening your eyes, mentally go over all the corners individually for a few seconds only. Then blinking for a few times rapidly at the letter on the chart, close your eyes again quickly and follow this process with other letters also.

Another similar exercise while palming is to try having clear mental pictures of the white space inside letters by following their outlines mentally, and noticing the sharp contrast of the white colour against the black letter. People with myopia (short-sightedness) are inclined to view this as a white letter with a black centre, and regular practice of deliberately changing the white and black background and letter is helpful.

Specific ideas of distant view and movement are of great benefit to successful relaxation while palming. Mentally picture a country that is stretching far away. In the distance visualise a cloud of dust gathering, suggesting the movement of a car advancing towards you, becoming visible as a tiny speck that gets larger as it gets nearer to you, then passes you in a rush.

Children especially need to be guided in imagination while palming, and the results are astonishingly wonderful and beneficial. Adults can imagine taking a stroll into the countryside while palming, observing all the things around them as they walk – trees, flowers, animals, vehicles, houses, birds, people, etc.

Palming benefits by acting as an antidote to acidity, since light-exposed retina becomes acidic.

Swaying

It is a truism that stationary objects that are nearby, will appear to move in the opposite direction to your own movement. For example, when a train carrying you moves at some speed, all that you view outside seems to be moving in the opposite direction at the same speed. This is an illusion which is evident in varying degrees under all circumstances in which we move.

When we move around in a room, the objects will appear to shift and alter their position either to the left or the right of us. This again, is just an illusion, for it is we who move, and not the objects.

Swaying and swinging exercises can be one of the most valuable and extensive aids to sight and general relaxation of the nerves and body. The sense of physical relaxation is easily achieved by rhythmic exercises, just like a rocking-chair has a soothing effect on the body.

Jaded and tensed nerves do not respond well to mental discipline, but will readily respond to simple physical rhythmic movement. Most of the swaying exercises are invariably done with the eyes closed, so that the visual picture is shut out and the sensitive nerves are relaxed.

Swaying exercises can be done sitting or standing, though swaying whilst standing is more advantageous as there is more balance on the feet, and more rhythm when the whole body is brought into play. Each individual may take his/her own time with swaying exercises to gain the sense of relaxation of the body, nerves and mind.

It is better to devote a few minutes to one form of exercise and then shift to another, rather than stick to a long continued attempt in any one particular exercise.

Exercise 1

- Stand comfortably with your feet a few inches apart from each other, hands hanging loosely at the sides, or clasped loosely in front.

- Sway the whole body to one side, say about nine inches to one foot from the body, so that the body weight is on one foot.
- Sway back to the original position, with the body weight now on the other foot.
- Ensure that the feet are firmly placed on the ground.
- Do not bend at the hips or neck, but make sure that the head, shoulders and hips all move together.
- The swaying time should not be less than one and a half to two seconds for each side.
- Practise this for a few minutes till you get the easy sense of physical balance, then close your eyes and try it again and again till you feel the same easy balance with your eyes open or closed.

Exercise 2

- Hang a chart or picture at one end of the room focusing good light upon it.
- Place a table in the middle of the room, and place an object having a width of 2-3 inches on it, tall enough to be in front of the chart.

- Stand at the other end of the room so that the object on the table is in your line of vision with the middle of the chart.
- Watch the chart and sway slowly to the left for a few inches (your view of the chart will be partly obscured by the object on the table).
- As you sway to the left, the chart will now be fully visible, with the object appearing to the right of the chart.
- Sway to your right, and this time the object will appear to be on the left side of the chart.
- As you sway rhythmically, the object on the table will appear alternately to cross the chart to the opposite side.
- You can either imagine the chart crossing behind the object, or the object moving in front of the chart – the sole purpose being to be conscious of the movement of the two objects in relation to your own movement.
- Now close your eyes, and imagine the movement of the objects while you sway to the left and right.
- Without altering your speed or rhythm, gradually shorten the distance of swaying, until the

movement gradually decreases without actually coming to a standstill.

- You will notice that the objects appear to move relatively less, and just proportionate to your own movement.
- Increase the distance of swaying again to nine inches or one foot till you can easily imagine and distinguish the alteration in distance.
- You may vary the exercise by hanging an object on a string from a light placed on the centre of the room, in line with a picture on one of the walls.
- While travelling in a vehicle, frequently close your eyes, and assess the speed at which you are travelling, visualising images of buildings, trees, people, vehicles, etc passing you.
- While walking, appreciate the rhythm and sway of the body from side to side with each step, conscious of the buildings, pavement, etc appearing to sway in the opposite direction.

Exercise 3

- Sit comfortably in a chair in the middle of a room, facing a chart on a wall.

- Hold the fingertips of one hand about a foot from your face, and in line with the middle of the chart.
- You can support your elbow with the help of the other hand.
- Turn your head very slowly to the left, and your hand will appear to move from the middle of the chart over to the right at just the same speed.
- Close your eyes and visualise the same relative movement of the hand across the chart.
- Practise mentally focusing on the hand at near distance and changing the focus to the chart at long distance, being conscious of the objects moving as you move.

Exercise 4

- Hold a book in front of you about a foot away.
- Hold a finger of the other hand in between your face and the book.
- Notice the finger moving in the opposite direction as you move your head even slightly.
- Practise this exercise mentally for a few minutes till you feel the finger swaying to and fro across the book as you turn your head to either side.

Exercise 5

- Take a convenient-sized cardboard, and make a hole in the centre about three inches in diameter.
- Keep this flat against an open page of a book.
- As you move the card along the line to the right, it will appear as though the words are travelling to the left.
- The effect is more noticeable if you practise it with one eye at a time.
- This exercise is most beneficial in treating presbyopia (a defect increasing with age).

Long swing

In swaying, a simple movement of the body or head alone is done, merely from side to side without turning the body at all, while in the long swing, the whole body is turned. The objective of the swing is to secure an increased sense of balance and poise, an easy rhythmic physical movement while the mind appreciates the apparent movement in an opposite direction of still objects in the background.

The swing is preferred to the sway as it facilitates a greater degree of physical movement. Apart from its utility in eyesight training, it is specifically useful in some cases of insomnia.

Exercise

- Stand relaxed with feet about a foot apart, hands hanging loosely by the sides, or clasped lightly in front, facing a wall.
- Slowly turn the whole body, shoulders and head together, to the right, by raising the left heel and turning it outward, until the shoulders and head are facing the wall on the right – a movement of 90 degrees.
- Now revert to the original position, lowering the heel of the left foot.
- Continue turning left another 90 degrees, this time raising the heel of the right foot outward.
- Make this whole movement continuous through a complete half circle (180 degrees) without a pause or a jerk.
- Notice that as you swing, the still objects appear to slide past in an opposite direction.
- Ensure that your swing is restricted to 90 degrees on either side, and not exceeding it.

- Also make sure that the foot, on the side to which you are swinging, remains firmly fixed on the ground, while only the heel of the other foot is raised and turned outward.
- When you transfer the weight from one foot to another, it should be done just when you are facing the wall.
- A good rhythm of one and a half to two seconds for each side is beneficial.

Variable sway

Make three charts with similar lettering on each and hang these at various distances – for example, 3 ft, 6 ft and 9 ft – away from you so that all three charts are visible and not overlapping each other.

- Sway slowly in a rhythmic and easy manner.
- Notice how the cards appear to overlap and separate alternately as you sway from side to side.
- While swaying, look at one of the letters on the nearest chart which appears to be the clearest to the eye.

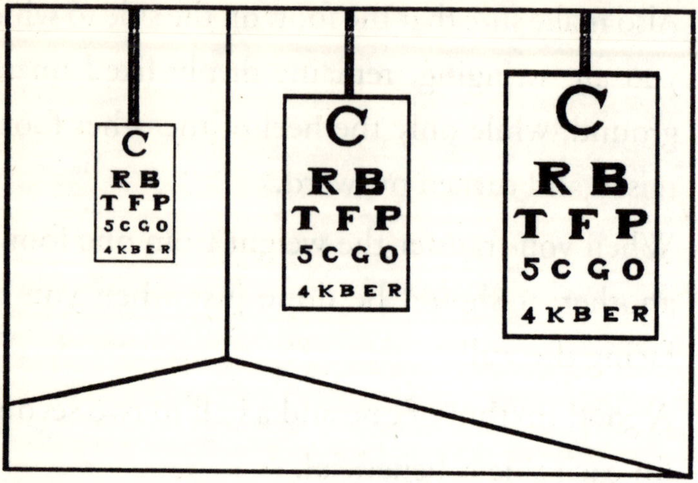

Figure 8

- Close your eyes, visualising the image of the chart and the letter as they seemingly move in the opposite direction as you sway.
- Open your eyes and look at the same letter on all the three charts in succession, beginning from the nearest.
- Repeat the same with the other letters.
- Practise with each eye separately and alternately, and then with both the eyes together.
- With this practise, both young and old can improve their distant sight.

Aids to Vision

When we see, there are certain imprints etched in our minds. These are usually associated with our memories and a result, affect our interpretation of these prints.

This factor is mainly responsible for many types of illusions and disorders of vision, for instance, a bedouin will naturally see distant objects better than others, as a habit and by practice, his mind gets used to judge distance. Most often our perception becomes associated with accustomed ways of seeing objects which we mentally interpret in a stereotyped form instead of in true perspective. For example, when we take the letter S or number 8, we are not wholly conscious of a difference in the size of the upper and lower parts of them till we invert them.

S S S S	S S S S
8 8 8 8	8 8 8 8

True perception then is influenced by images from the memory which is the ability to recall an impression which must have been made upon the mind.

The clearer and more detailed the visual image, the stronger will be the mental impression, and the easier it will be to remember. It is important therefore that the mind, memory or imagination be trained with the eye – the image focused onto the retina is not sight, but becomes so when the mind, memory or imagination reconstructs the object. In other words, the image needs to be visualised before we are conscious of what we see. Over-exposure and irritation of the retina in the eye is prevented either by closing the eyelid or by immediately and simultaneously visualising the picture.

Very often, the eyes are open, and the image of whatever is in the area of vision is mechanically projected onto the retina, but the visual perceptions made by the stimulation of the nerve-ends on the retina do not excite attention – this is absent-mindedness, or day-dreaming, or being preoccupied or having a vacant stare. A well-coordinated action between the mind and eye is essential – the eye without the mind will not interpret the image that is created, and the mind without the eye can only recall a past image, but not what you are seeing at present.

It is advisable to close the eyes and stop thinking instead of letting any image to be focused on the retina and wasting energy.

Whatever we may judge by gesture or intonation of voice, only the eyes can convey the self-expression on the face of a person, they being called aptly the 'windows of the soul'.

The problem of the backward child results from untrained coordination between the mind and eye, and he needs to be guided into being aware of what he is seeing. Macular development therefore appears to be coincident with the capacity of thought power.

Visual Coordination

Putting vividly before the mind's eye the object you wish to see, helps the eye to see that object.

Always remember that visualising images with the eyes shut follows the same law of macular vision as ordinary seeing does.

Exercise 1

- Place a large chart in good light, free from glare or reflection.
- Stand at a distance from where several large letters are clear and distinct.
- Select a letter from the chart, close your eyes and visualise it.
- If you focus on the white space inside the letter, for instance, the letter A, and try to see the whole letter equally clearly at once, parts of it will appear grey, and not clearly black.

- If you allow the mental focus to shift around the letter, it will appear more black, with the edges clearer and sharper, and the white space inside the letter appearing whiter.
- Though this is a natural illusion, it should be encouraged for improving your sight.
- The clearer and blacker your mental impression of the letter becomes, the clearer and whiter in contrast will be the background, especially the white space inside the letter.

Exercise 2

- Again close your eyes and visualise the letter you have selected.
- Now divide it vertically into equal halves.
- Keep your mental focus upon one half of the letter only, merely ignoring the other half, but not trying to shut it out completely.
- Then focus on the left half of the letter, and slowly move it down and up, as if tracing its outline, and its clear edges.
- As you keep doing this, this half of the letter will appear blacker and clearer than the other half.

- Change your focus to the other half of the letter now, and similarly move it down and up till you get the same effect.
- It is easier to visualise one part of the letter at a time than to endeavour to keep the whole letter in focus at once.

Exercise 3

- Now try the same with another letter, say the letter, B.
- First look at the large letter from a distance from where it is conveniently visible.
- Close your eyes and visualise it, keeping the focus moving over the line and curves of the letter.
- While visualising, note the white spaces within the letter, each looking like the letter D.
- Now concentrate only on the upper half of the letter, ignoring the lower half, and you will notice that this half appears to be clearer.
- Then focus on the white space in the lower half of the letter.
- You cannot visualise an equally clear picture of both the white spaces at the same time unless

you imagine the whole letter to be at some distance away from you.

Exercise 4

- Place a coin each on the two white spaces of the letter B.
- Glancing at both of them at the same time, you will be able to identify them as two separate coins, but will be unable to read the date on each of them without shifting the focus from one to the other.

Exercise 5

- With eyes closed, slowly walk backwards from the chart, and visualise the letter moving farther away in the distance.
- After each step backwards, stop, blink a few times quickly while watching the letter, close your eyes and visualise it getting slightly smaller as you move away from the chart.
- Take another step backward, and continue the process of blinking and moving backward, till the two white space no longer look like the letter D but appear as mere white dots.

Exercise 6

- Hang a few charts of equal size along each railing of a fence.
- Glance at a letter on the nearest chart, close your eyes, and visualise it clearly.
- Open your eyes and glance at the same letter on the next chart, and allow your focus to shift around the letter, seeing it clearly.
- Continue this process along the fence, and it will become evident that the nearer ones will be clear, and the others will appear smaller and smaller until lost to the mind's eye.

Illusions of Sight

- Only part of what we see comes to the eye from the object, while the remainder comes from the visual sense in the brain where past experiences of having seen similar objects before, are stored.
- It is therefore necessary to practise seeing things in a new perspective.
- By stimulating the imagination, visual judgement and attention, we improve our vision.

Illusion 1

- The horizontal lines in the two sets of drawings are parallel.
- To prove this, tilt the page sideways and look along the lines from the edge.
- When you again look at them directly, try and visualise them as parallel.

- This is interpreted only in length and breath, the unusual being the contrasting lines of angle and direction.
- The best and easiest way of using this illustration is to observe the illusion first with one eye, then with the other, and finally with both eyes together – a good practice for the cultivation of macular vision.

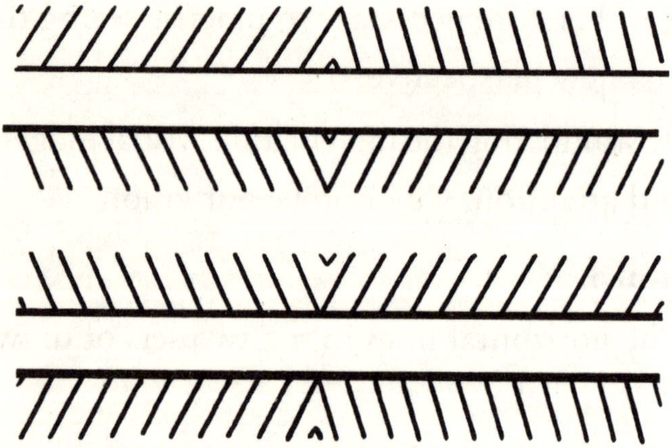

Figure 9

Illusion 2

- The outline of the square in each of the two drawings appears distorted.
- To prove that they are squares, slowly tilt the page backwards till it is almost horizontal again – 180 degrees.

- Now notice that they are actually squares.
- When you revert to the original position, appreciate them as squares.

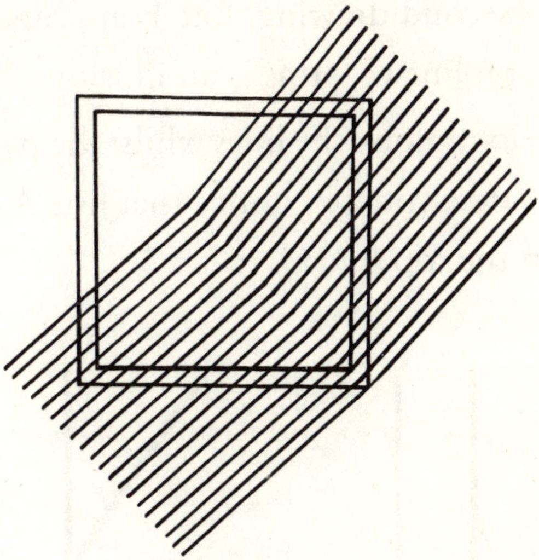

Figure 10

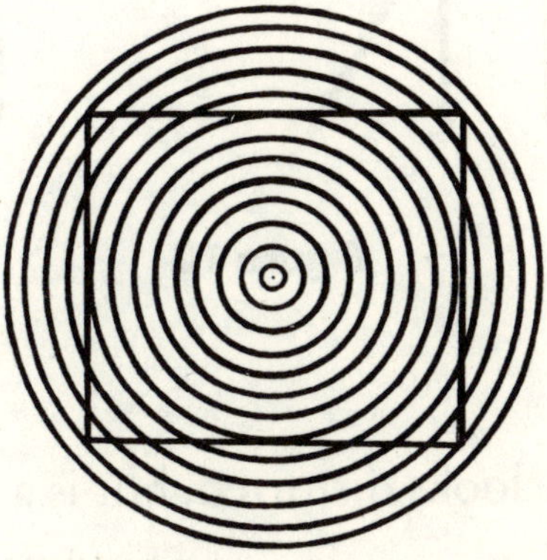

Figure 11

Illusion 3

- In the first drawing, the oblique lines would meet on the vertical line.
- In the second drawing, line B appears to extend above on line C – this is an illusion.
- If you look along the lines whilst the page is tilted backwards, you will notice that line A continues to run the top line C.

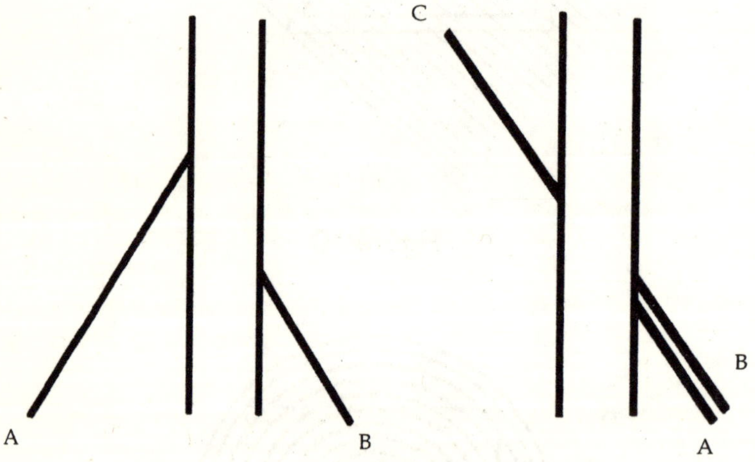

Figure 12

Illusion 4

- The circle looks distorted, but is a perfect round.
- It is interesting to notice the difficulty which is sometimes experienced in changing the mental

focus, even when it is known what to look for in the illusion.

- The ability to change the mental focus rapidly improves with practice.

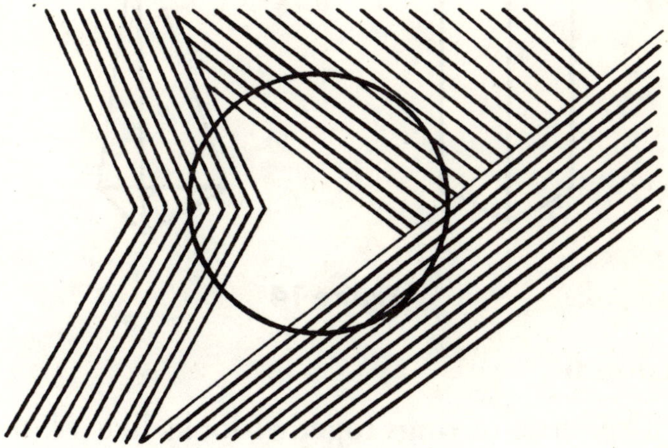

Figure 13

Illusion 5

- The first drawing can be a book or card folded down the centre.
- It looks at one angle as if it is the outside cover of the book.
- It also looks like the inner pages of a book.

- When you see the second drawing, it looks like a pyramid standing on its base, or as leaning backwards, with its base fully visible.

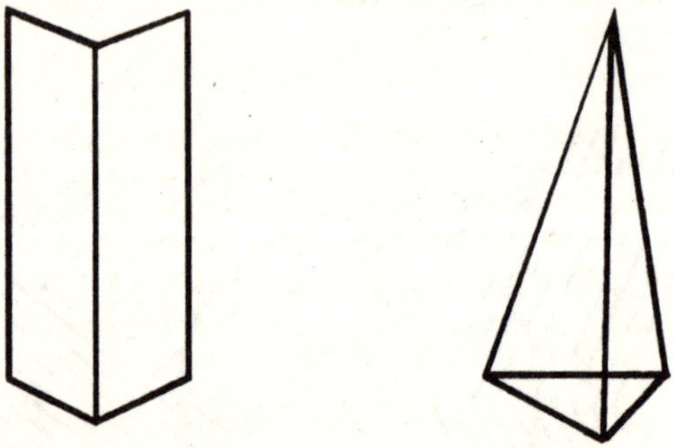

Figure 14

Illusion 6

- The series of rings together looks like a kind of skeleton tube.
- If you focus on either of the end circles, it will appear that the near end of the tube is either on the left or on the right.

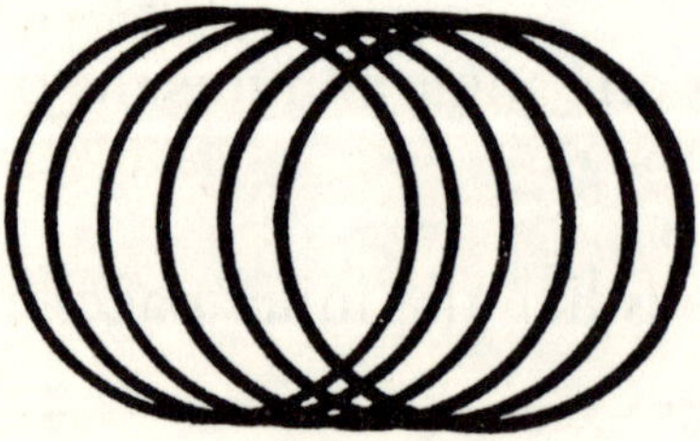

Figure 15

Illusion 7

- At first glance the drawing looks like a staircase being looked at diagonally from the top.
- A closer and focused look presents another view – as if one is looking at the stairs from underneath.
- This will prove more difficult to many people to appreciate.

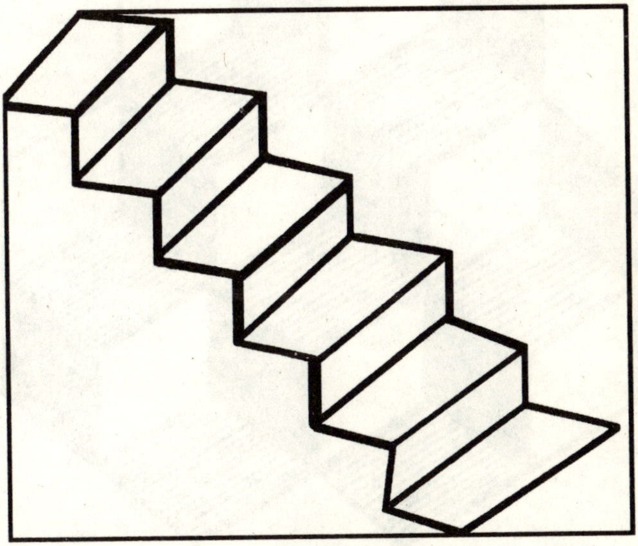

Figure 16

Illusion 8

- When you view this drawing, you will normally see six cubes at first glance.
- If you look carefully, another perspective offers seven cubes.

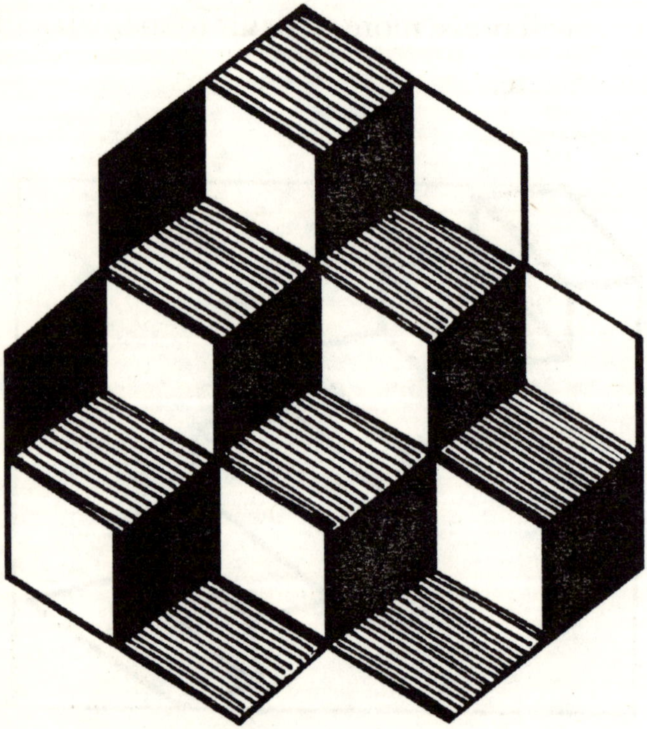

Figure 17

Myopia and Its Treatment

When the eye is in a relaxed state and a distant object forms an image in front of, and not on, the retina, this is a state of myopia, or short-sightedness. The image quite literally falls short of the screen-receptor.

A myopic eye has difficulty in reducing its power when focused on distant objects, but as the divergence of light increases, the image will fall on the retina, making it possible for the eye to see the object clearly.

The inability to see may be caused by either the eyeball being too long from back to front (axial –

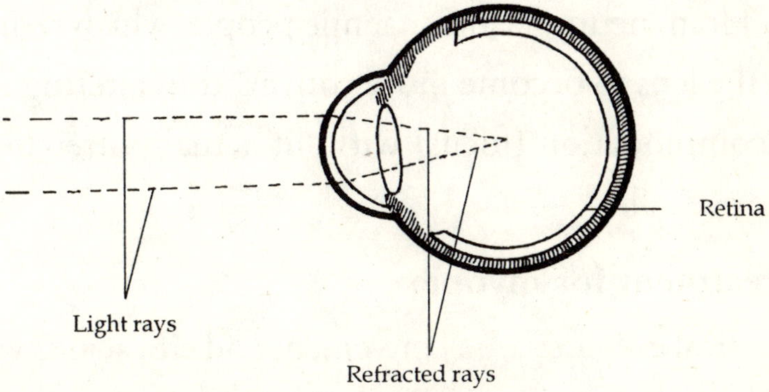

Figure 18

myopia), or, if the eyeball is of normal shape, then the refractive power is too great (refractive or index myopia).

Myopic people can see nearby objects quite distinctly, but by looking close to see clearly, they strain excessively the power of convergence leading to varying forms of ocular congestion.

In children particularly, a quite common peril following the excessive strain of myopia, is a varied form of squint. Myopia needs special care, for, if neglected, it may lead to dire consequences like haemorrhage, detachment of the retina, floating specks, choroidal atrophy, etc.

In accommodative myopia, the ciliary muscle, composed of involuntary muscle fibres, is apt to develop into a state of lens contraction, especially in children, neurotic and anaemic people, which results in the lens to become more convex, thus altering the accommodation (focus) without actually stretching the eyeball.

Treatment for myopia

Physical exercises are a convenient and efficacious way of stimulating the metabolic processes.

- Myopics should hold their head normally erect and get rid of stooping.
- Blink consistently under all conditions.
- Close your eyes while engrossed in thinking.
- Encourage the frequent use of each eye separately both for near and distant vision.
- Move your focus rapidly and continuously as if looking at some detail or tracing outlines.
- When objects are not clearly visible, instead of straining to see them clearly, make use of flashing glances and momentarily closing of eyes.
- For reading, change the distance frequently both nearer and farther away.
- Swaying and swinging, especially the long swing, help in treating myopia.
- Central fixation exercises also help in myopic cases.
- Watching the sun rise early in the morning helps in the stimulation of the pituitary gland, which, in a way, has an effect on the eyes.

Long-sightedness and Astigmatism: Their Treatment

Long sight occurs when the optical power of the whole eye is too weak to bring the image on to the retina, but instead projects it some distance beyond.

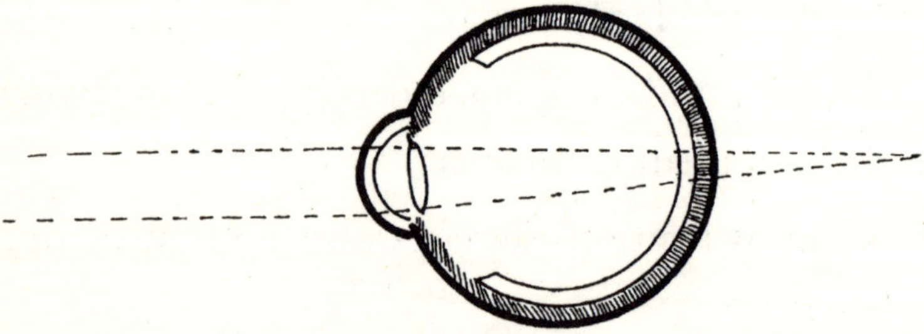

Figure 19

A person suffering from long sight (also called hyperopia or hypermetropia), whilst able to focus easily on distant objects, may find it more difficult to see nearby objects effortlessly, and consequently develop symptoms of eye-strain. The difference between myopia and hypermetropia is that the light rays, in the form of an image, do not reach the retina until after they have come to a focus in short-sighted people, but in long-sighted people, they reach the retina before they come to a focus.

Long sight is more often caused by the eyeball being relatively too short from front to back (axial-Hypermetropia), or from an abnormal refractive index of the cornea, lens, aqueous or vitreous humour. Long sight strains normally result in red and inflamed eyelids, giddiness and discomfort while working.

In old age, presbyopia (old age sight) sets in, where the eyes normally fail to accommodate with ageing. In presbyopia, with advancing years, the vision matter gets blurred and there is a tendency to rub the eyes and look into the distance to ease tiredness.

Treatment for longsightedness

- Relax the eyes by closing them frequently, with occasional palming.

- Allow flexibility to continue by blinking and exercising the ocular muscles by movements of the eyeballs, alternating the focus near and far.
- Bathe the closed eyes a few times daily.
- The practice of alternate contraction and dilation of the pupil by letting the eyes get accustomed to the dark in a darkened room with blinds for half a minute. Then pulling the blind aside and looking at the light for a few seconds, can prove to be very beneficial for myopic people.
- Close your eyes and visualise some words typed in black on a white page. Then open the eyes and read as long as the type is seen black, and close your eyes again when the typed words blur.
- Hold some reading material and shake it quickly while watching it for a few seconds. Then hold it still and see, how the type appears clear, before blurring again. Repeat this again, for it is a quick method of gaining benefit.
- All reading may be done at a little closer range than normal, not close enough to make the reading faint, but always a little nearer than one would normally hold it – beginning with the

larger type, proceeding to smaller type and relaxing the eyes every few lines looking into the distance.

- You can alternate with the left and right eye for each paragraph, and at times use both eyes for reading.
- Use the card with the large hole for reading few lines in large type, and gradually shifting to smaller type at a close distance that is convenient – this will relieve the tendency of feeling restrained by the small amount of vision which the hole imposes.
- A little coaxing can overcome old age problem of poor sight by this exercise – place a card of small type letters in good light. Relax your eyes by palming, visualising the lines of the small, black print against the whiteness of the spaces between the lines. Open your eyes, blink quickly a few times at the print, moving it alternately nearer and farther from the eyes, and notice the contrast of black lines and white spaces. Look into the distance for a few seconds, then back to the print. Keep on repeating the exercise merely allowing

an occasional word to come up clear at once, and soon some of the print will become clear.

Astigmatism

This is an eye defect, usually in the cornea, which prevents the eye from focusing properly, and results in distorted or blurred vision.

Most cases of astigmatism are of simple, vertical or horizontal type. This is caused by unequal tension of the upper and lower recti muscles as opposed to the muscles on either side, resulting in a relative flattening of the eye in one meridian. A scar on the cornea after an accident or operation can be responsible for astigmatism, or it may be hereditary.

Treatment for astigmatism

- A person having astigmatism must get rid of the bad habit of staring, and especially making an effort to see things.
- Close your eyes while thinking about something.
- Palming and bathing of the eyes also prove to be beneficial.
- Occasionally shut your eyes for a few times while exercising and relax.

- Roll your eyeballs slowly in different directions, without straining, a few times to restore flexibility.
- Swaying exercises are helpful in relieving the tensed eye muscles.

Squint and Amblyopia

Squint, also known as strabismus, is a condition in which both eyes fail to focus on the same spot at the same time.

When one or both eyes are turned in towards the nose, the disorder is called convergent strabismus, or cross-eye. When one or both eyes turn outwards towards the temples, the condition is known as divergent strabismus.

Squint is due to some abnormality of the extrinsic muscles.

The brain blends or fuses together the individual image of each eye, so that we are conscious of only one image.

Very often the image of one eye is comparatively less distinct than that of the other eye, and this is one of the common causes which interferes with perfect vision, or binocular vision. Sometimes, when the images appear to be unequal to the eyes, the brain is unable to blend them together, and hence ignores the weaker and diffused image. As a result, the sight of the weaker eyes gets suppressed, leading to amblyopia or blurred vision. Inequality in the muscle pull of the eyes, known as muscular imbalance, gives rise to pain and headache, due to latent squint, where the squint is not visible as the sense of fusion of muscles is still powerful enough to keep the focus of the eyes straight.

The definite or manifest squint is the form commonly seen, and cannot ordinarily be corrected.

Treatment for squint

- Eliminating strain factors leads to successful treatment of squints.
- Muscular flexibility should be cultivated.
- In order to avoid strain to the eyes, it is advisable to avoid harsh noises, shocks, sudden changes, distractions, despondency and fatigue.
- Avoid staring, as it is one of the most fertile sources of squint.
- It is beneficial to exercise the weaker eye frequently by covering the other eye while

exercising, so as to avoid the weaker eye from becoming amblyopic.

- For muscular flexibility, blink frequently in an easy manner without strain.
- Roll the eyes in all directions in a gentle manner.
- Another exercise for correcting squint is to close or cover one eye, and with the other eye, look at your fingertip (kept at a distance of about one foot from the face), then at something in the distance, then back at the fingertip, thus alternating the focus near and far ten times, about two seconds each way. Repeat this with the other eye, and then with both the eyes.
- The same exercise can later be done by bringing the fingertip closer to your nose, stopping at the point where both eyes fail to follow it together, and repeating again from a foot away.
- Read a book at the ordinary distance, and gradually bring it closer to the eyes until the print appears blurred, then move it back to the original distance.
- When only one eye has a squint, cover the other eye, and make the affected eye follow the finger

or object held at arm's outwards ten or twenty times, repeating it often.

Eye Diseases and Disorders

Certain conditions of the eye disorders, like detachment of the retina, need radical local measures, whereas others such as atrophy of the optic nerve, choroiditis and retinitis need prolonged treatment.

Many people are averse to radical operative treatment, preferring measures of sensible nature cure instead.

Detachment of the retina

This means a separation of some part of the retina from the choroid to which it is normally attached, resulting in distorted or loss of vision. This could be due to an accidental blow to the eye, a growth, or acute degree of myopia.

Only some definite strain will detach the retina wholly or partially, and hence one having a high degree of myopia should refrain from such violent games as football. Such a person should not lift heavy weight, stoop or raise with undue suddenness; swimming and diving should be avoided, and opening the eyes under water should be avoided. In such cases, palming is a good practice to relax the eye muscles.

Retinitis and choroiditis

These are generally understood to be due to some disease of the general system such as syphilis, diabetes, kidney problem, etc.

A natural way to seek cure for these is to follow a complete and systematic food reform under a competent adviser, and to practice relaxation exercises given in this book.

Cataract

This is a clouded condition of the lens of the eye, which causes blurred vision.

Over-exposure of the eyes to heat, x-rays, nuclear radiation, an injury, or a disease such as diabetes, may cause cataracts, in which one or both eyes may get affected. Palming, swaying and visualising are beneficial for those having cataract. Wearing sun glasses when stepping out into the hot sunny weather would help.

Diet is again an important factor, and care should be taken to avoid acid-forming foods such as excess of fish, meat and chicken, eggs and most of the nuts. Instead, have more of milk, fresh fruit and vegetables, and plenty of water.

Close your eyes and wash them frequently with warm or cold water.

Alternate contraction and dilation of the pupil is also helpful.

Glaucoma

This is a disorder of the eyes caused by increased pressure of fluid within the eyeballs, and, if untreated, can lead to blindness. Much can be done by judicious dieting by avoiding organic ingredients like albumin, and excessive mineral salts.

- Palming provides much relief.
- Recalling easy, clear picture is valuable.
- Swaying gently has therapeutic benefits.
- The long swing before retiring to bed also helps.

Floating specks

These are tiny opacities floating in the vitreous humour of the eye that assume various shapes like flakes, strings of leads, noodle-like strings, etc, especially during attacks of biliousness, and more often in the myopics.

- General toning up of health is essential.
- Avoid staring and straining the eyes.
- Palming and swaying are definitely beneficial.

Glare

Glare strain can be due to sensitiveness to light, staring and straining to focus properly, sudden shift from darkness into bright light, the glare reflected from shiny or white surfaces, over-exposed and unshaded artificial lights, or the glaring headlights of a car on a dark night.

The intolerance of light by the eyes is known as photophobia, and is due to the effects of special bands of the light spectrum, and due to an undue sensitiveness of the retina.

- Bathe the closed eyes with water to soothe the optical nerves.
- Allow the eyes to gradually accustom to ordinary standards of light, and even to extra bright light by carefully sunbathing the closed eyes for a few minutes.

Styes

The stye is an inflammation of the hair follicles at the margin of the eyelid, caused by infection in one or more eyelash roots, or in the sebaceous glands. A small, hard area that is quite tender appears on the edge of the lid, and soon a cyst filled with pus rises in the middle.

Styes usually indicate both constitutional disorder and some refractive error, or strained use of the eye. Hygiene is necessary, and lukewarm bathing with a simple and approved disinfectant like boracic lotion helps.

- Avoid staring, and encourage blinking.
- Palming and cultivation of the habit of easy macular vision are beneficial.

Inflamed eyes

Inflamed eyes could be due to conjunctivitis or iritis, or due to some minor irritants.

In conjunctivitis, the conjunctiva or the membrane that lines the eyelids and covers the ball, becomes inflamed due to some bacteria or virus. The eyelids swell and tend to stick together, and there may be a pus-containing discharge. Eyes also get inflamed with measles, scarlet fever and chickenpox. Dust, smoke and smog can also lead to the eyes getting inflamed.

Rheumatism and syphilis predispose to iritis which is a chronic inflammation of the iris, the coloured part of the eye.

- Swaying and palming are the safest and most effacious exercises to help alleviate the inflammation.
- Application of cold fomentations in conjunctivitis and hot ones in iritis are comforting.
- Avoid bright light, exposure to dust and fumes, and nasal douches.

Nystagmus

This is constant involuntary oscillation of the eyeball, usually affecting both eyes.

It occurs as a congenital nervous disorder such as multiple sclerosis and Meniere's disease. Occupational nystagmus necessitates a total change of work and environment.

Excellent and permanent results can be obtained by regular practice of palming and swaying.

Ptosis

This is the drooping of the upper eyelid caused by a muscle weakness or paralysis, leading to interference with vision.

General exhaustion or hysteria can lead to ptosis of one eye. In the congenital form, the condition can be helped by tilting the head backwards, and also by wrinkling the forehead in an effort to use the temporal muscle.

Consistent palming and bathing the closed eyes with water frequently, provide excellent results.

Colour blindness

This is the condition in which a person is unable to distinguish between certain colours. For example, red from green, although blue-green and red-blue colour blindness are also common.

Colour blindness is a disorder, not a disease. Use of certain drugs, alcohol, tobacco, and jaundice can lead to colour blindness, but most often it is hereditary.

Apart from food reform and general toning up of the metabolic processes, palming and swaying should be carried out.